SPANLINGO SPANISH
ANATOMY CHARTS

ENGLISH TO SPANISH

WITH WORKBOOK & ANSWER KEYS

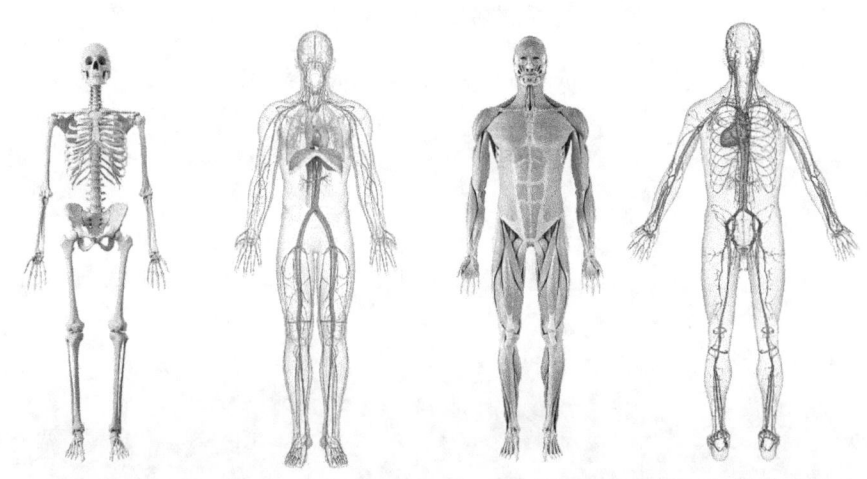

GEORGIA PATILIS

Charts by Tina Pavlatos

INDEX

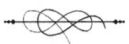

THE HEAD-LA CABEZA

The head, La cabeza

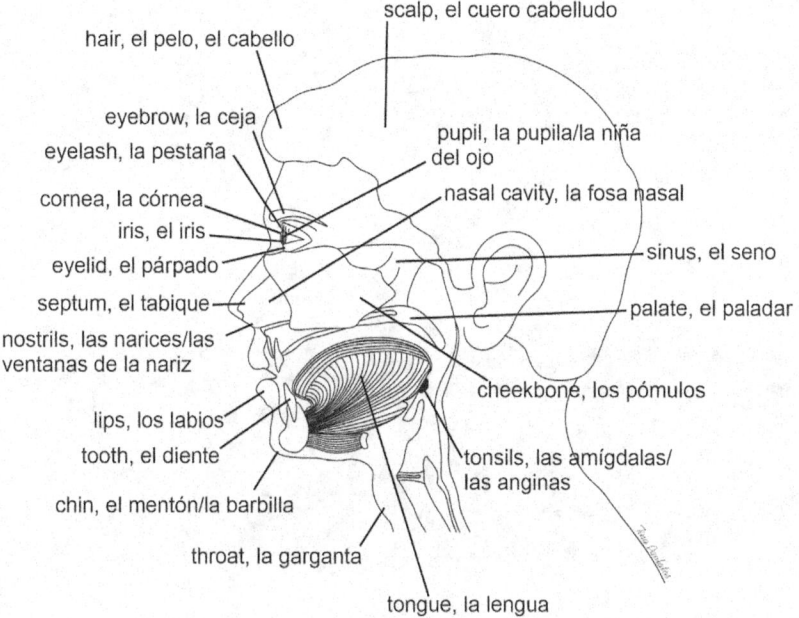

scalp, el cuero cabelludo

hair, el pelo, el cabello

eyebrow, la ceja
eyelash, la pestaña

pupil, la pupila/la niña del ojo

cornea, la córnea

nasal cavity, la fosa nasal

iris, el iris
eyelid, el párpado

sinus, el seno

septum, el tabique

palate, el paladar

nostrils, las narices/las ventanas de la nariz

lips, los labios

cheekbone, los pómulos

tooth, el diente

tonsils, las amígdalas/ las anginas

chin, el mentón/la barbilla

throat, la garganta

tongue, la lengua

THE MOUTH-LA BOCA

Mouth, Boca

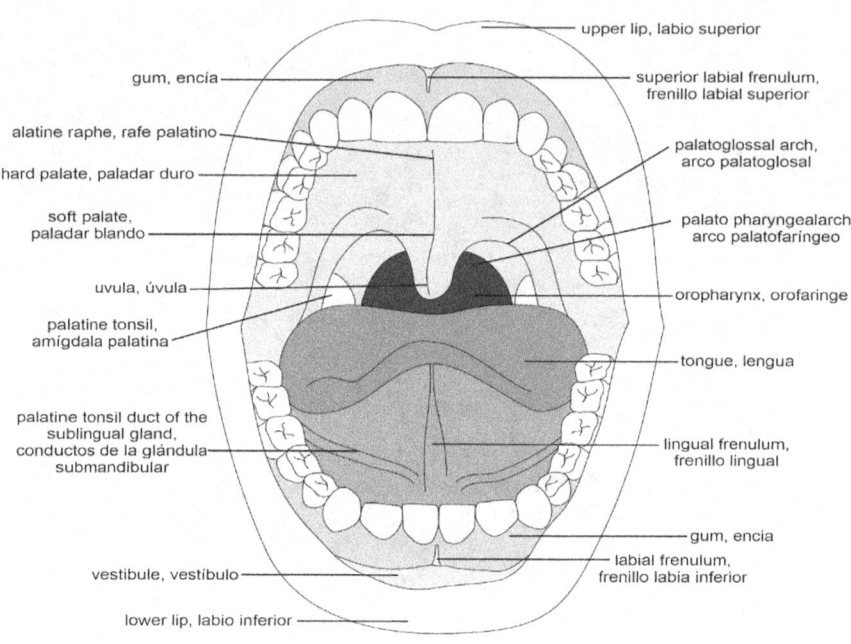

- upper lip, labio superior
- gum, encía
- superior labial frenulum, frenillo labial superior
- alatine raphe, rafe palatino
- palatoglossal arch, arco palatoglosal
- hard palate, paladar duro
- soft palate, paladar blando
- palato pharyngealarch, arco palatofaríngeo
- uvula, úvula
- oropharynx, orofaringe
- palatine tonsil, amígdala palatina
- tongue, lengua
- palatine tonsil duct of the sublingual gland, conductos de la glándula submandibular
- lingual frenulum, frenillo lingual
- gum, encia
- vestibule, vestíbulo
- labial frenulum, frenillo labia inferior
- lower lip, labio inferior

THE HUMAN BODY-EL CUERPO HUMANO

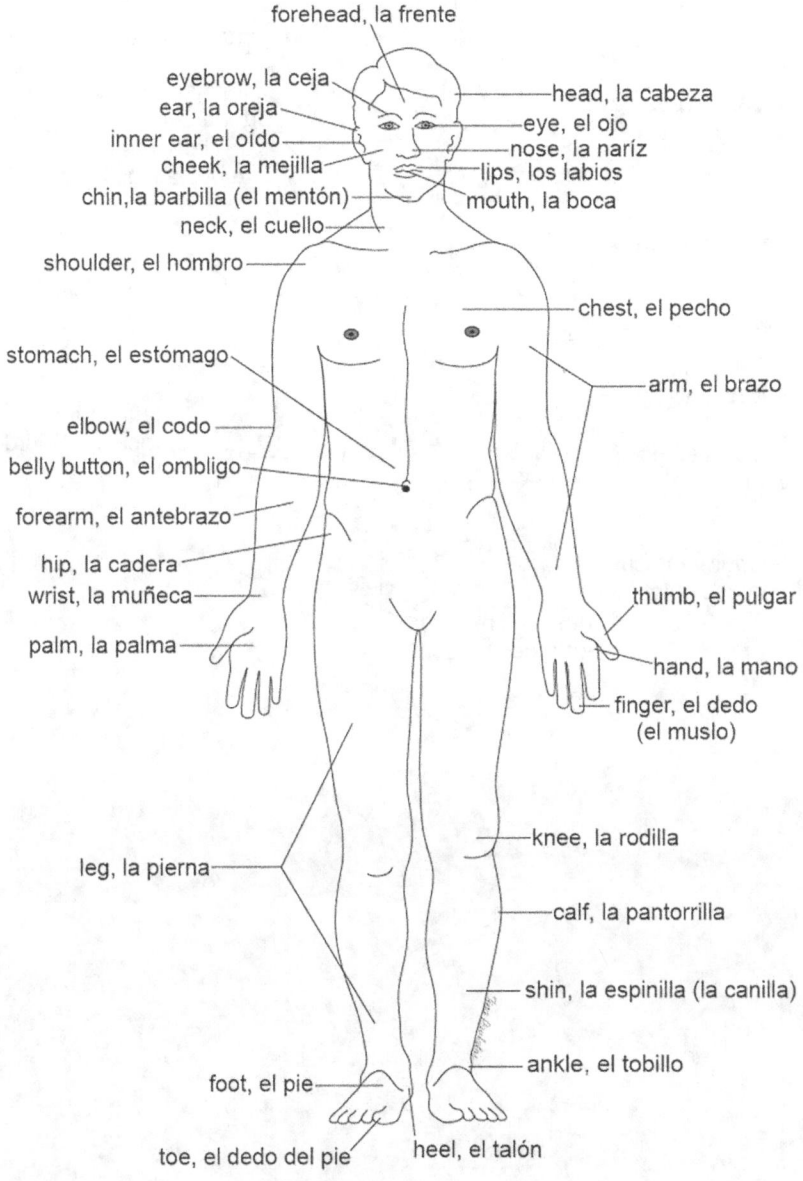

The human body, El cuerpo humano

forehead, la frente

eyebrow, la ceja
ear, la oreja
inner ear, el oído
cheek, la mejilla
chin, la barbilla (el mentón)
neck, el cuello

head, la cabeza
eye, el ojo
nose, la naríz
lips, los labios
mouth, la boca

shoulder, el hombro

chest, el pecho

stomach, el estómago

arm, el brazo

elbow, el codo
belly button, el ombligo

forearm, el antebrazo

hip, la cadera
wrist, la muñeca

thumb, el pulgar

palm, la palma

hand, la mano
finger, el dedo
(el muslo)

knee, la rodilla

leg, la pierna

calf, la pantorrilla

shin, la espinilla (la canilla)

ankle, el tobillo

foot, el pie

toe, el dedo del pie   heel, el talón

THE HEART-EL CORAZON

The heart, El corazón

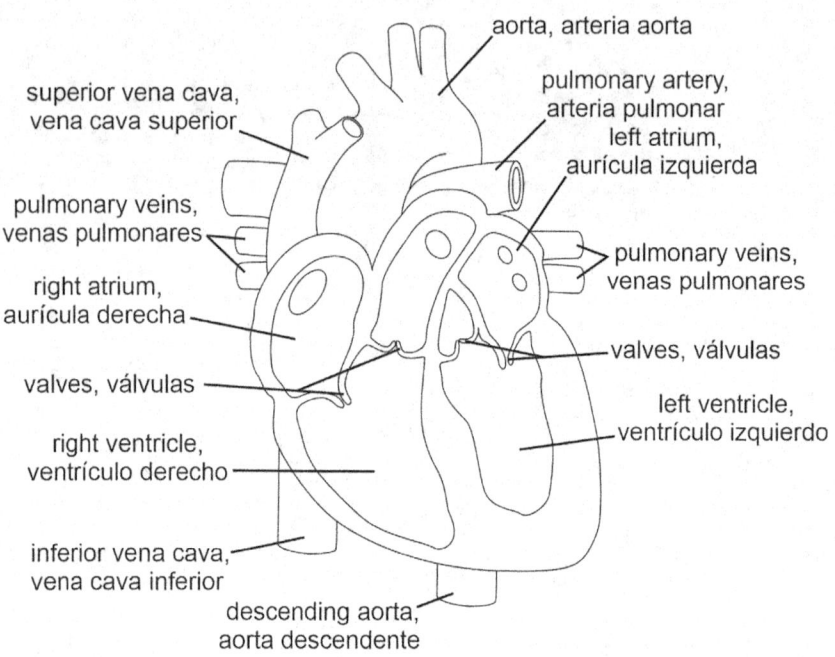

aorta, arteria aorta

superior vena cava,
vena cava superior

pulmonary artery,
arteria pulmonar
left atrium,
aurícula izquierda

pulmonary veins,
venas pulmonares

right atrium,
aurícula derecha

pulmonary veins,
venas pulmonares

valves, válvulas

valves, válvulas

left ventricle,
ventrículo izquierdo

right ventricle,
ventrículo derecho

inferior vena cava,
vena cava inferior

descending aorta,
aorta descendente

THE CIRCULATORY SYSTEM-EL SISTEMA CIRCULATORIO

Circulatory system, Sistema circulatorio

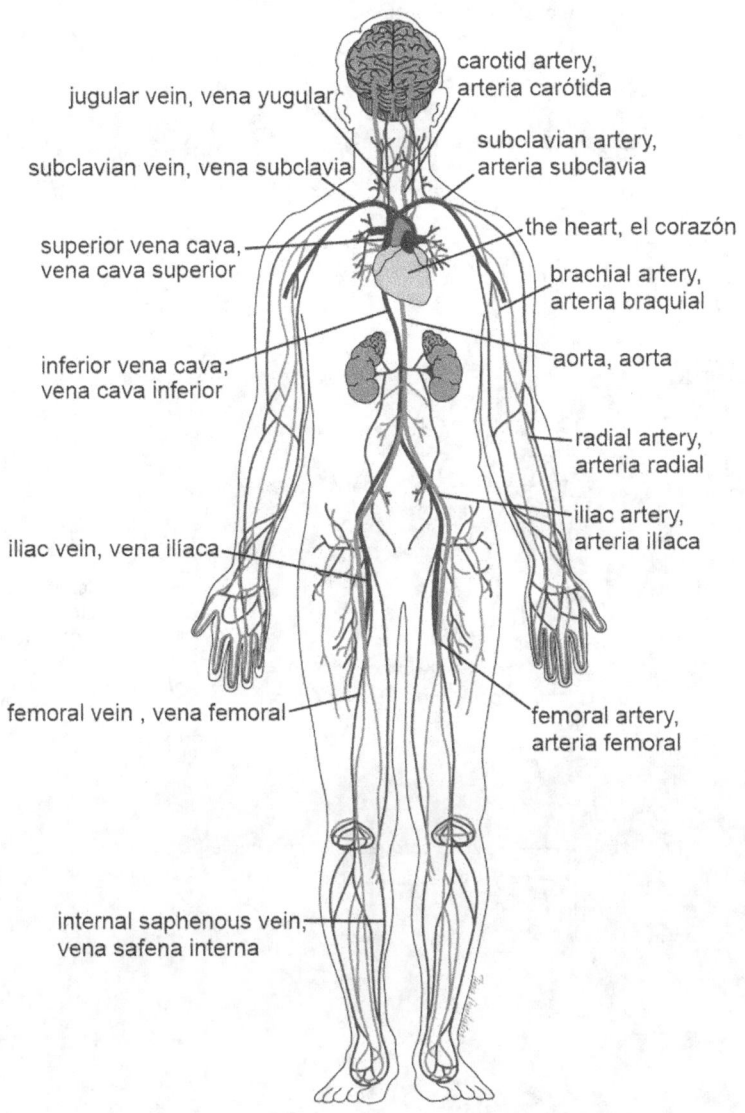

jugular vein, vena yugular

carotid artery, arteria carótida

subclavian vein, vena subclavia

subclavian artery, arteria subclavia

superior vena cava, vena cava superior

the heart, el corazón

brachial artery, arteria braquial

inferior vena cava, vena cava inferior

aorta, aorta

radial artery, arteria radial

iliac vein, vena ilíaca

iliac artery, arteria ilíaca

femoral vein , vena femoral

femoral artery, arteria femoral

internal saphenous vein, vena safena interna

THE NERVOUS SYSTEM-EL
SISTEMA NERVIOSO

The nervous system, El sistema nervioso

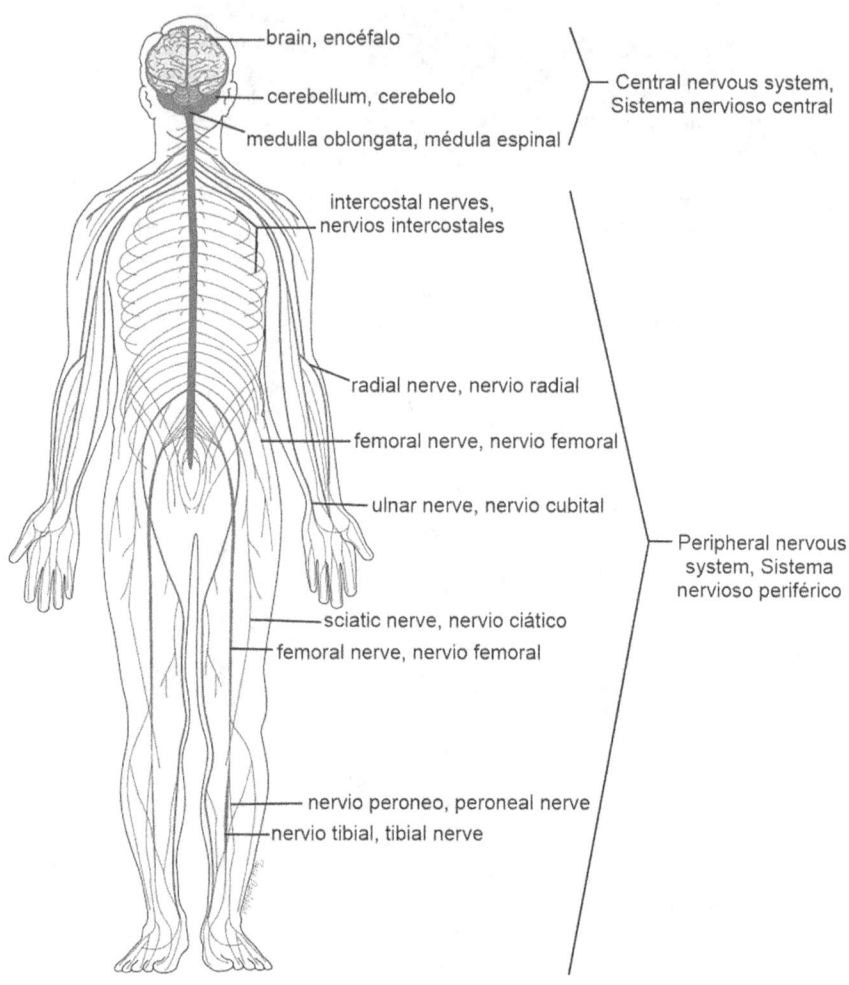

brain, encéfalo

cerebellum, cerebelo

medulla oblongata, médula espinal

Central nervous system,
Sistema nervioso central

intercostal nerves,
nervios intercostales

radial nerve, nervio radial

femoral nerve, nervio femoral

ulnar nerve, nervio cubital

Peripheral nervous
system, Sistema
nervioso periférico

sciatic nerve, nervio ciático
femoral nerve, nervio femoral

nervio peroneo, peroneal nerve
nervio tibial, tibial nerve

THE DIGESTIVE SYSTEM-EL SISTEMA DIGESTIVO

Digestive system, Aparato digestivo

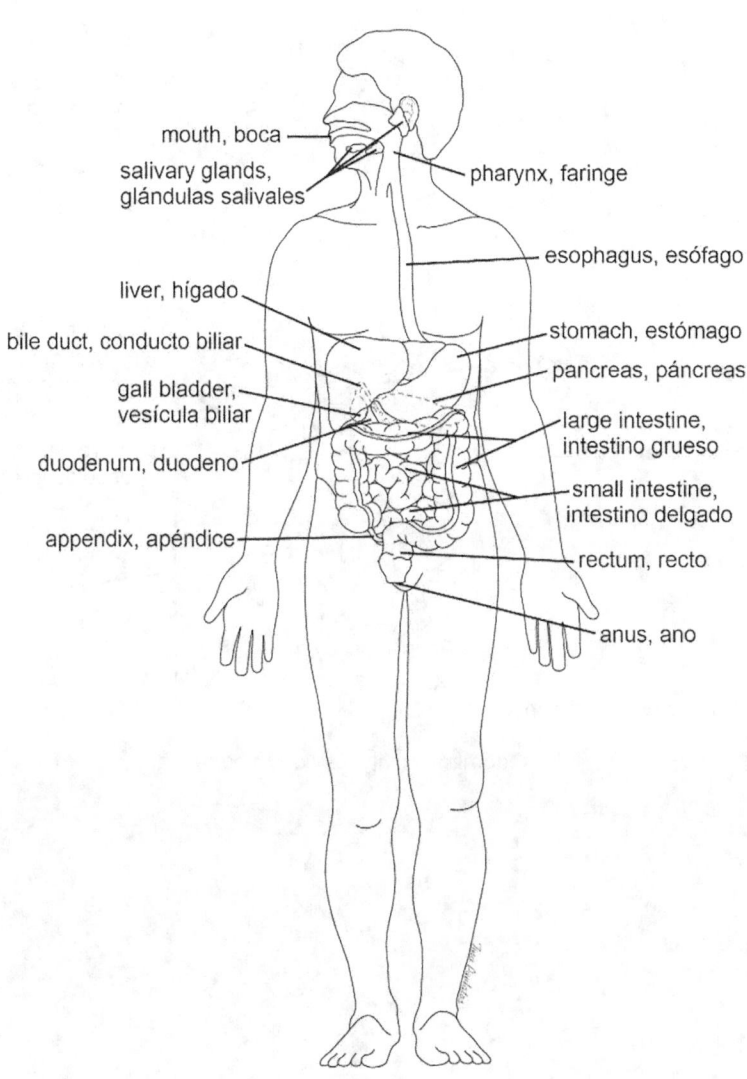

THE RESPIRATORY SYSTEM-EL SISTEMA RESPIRATORIO

The respiratory system, El sisterna respiratorio

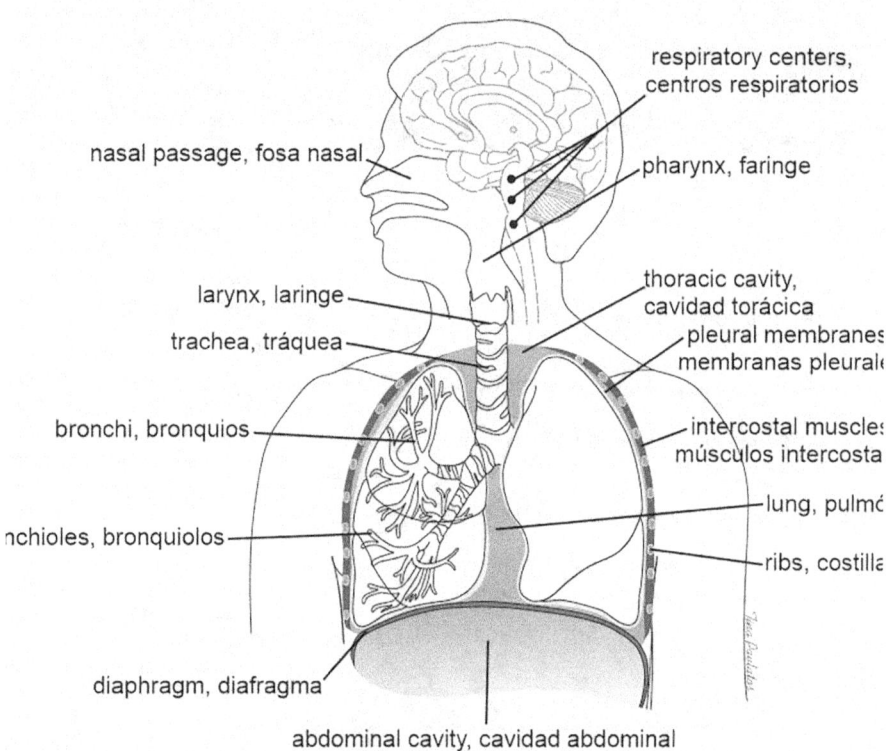

respiratory centers, centros respiratorios

nasal passage, fosa nasal

pharynx, faringe

larynx, laringe

trachea, tráquea

thoracic cavity, cavidad torácica

pleural membranes, membranas pleurale

bronchi, bronquios

intercostal muscles, músculos intercosta

nchioles, bronquiolos

lung, pulmó

ribs, costilla

diaphragm, diafragma

abdominal cavity, cavidad abdominal

THE SKELETAL SYSTEM-EL SISTEMA ESQUELETICO

The skeletal system, El sistema esquelético, (el sistema óseo)

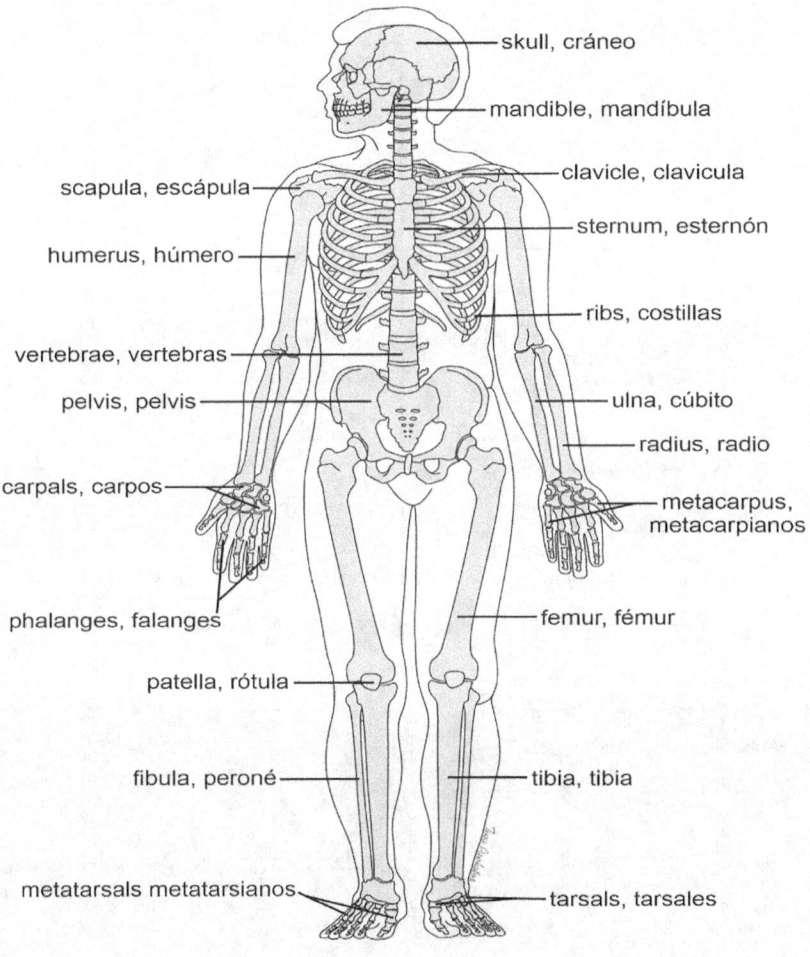

skull, cráneo

mandible, mandíbula

clavicle, clavicula

scapula, escápula

sternum, esternón

humerus, húmero

ribs, costillas

vertebrae, vertebras

pelvis, pelvis

ulna, cúbito

radius, radio

carpals, carpos

metacarpus, metacarpianos

phalanges, falanges

femur, fémur

patella, rótula

fibula, peroné

tibia, tibia

metatarsals metatarsianos

tarsals, tarsales

THE MUSCULAR SYSTEM-EL
SISTEMA MUSCULAR

The muscular system, El sistema muscular

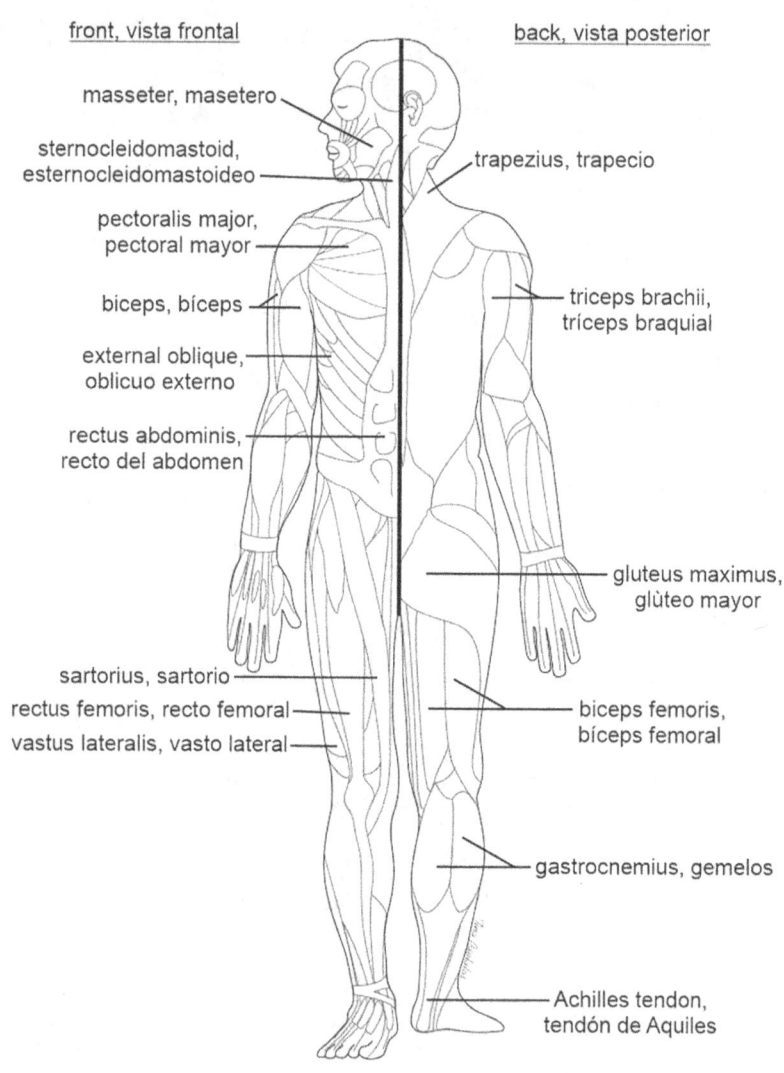

front, vista frontal

back, vista posterior

masseter, masetero

sternocleidomastoid,
esternocleidomastoideo

trapezius, trapecio

pectoralis major,
pectoral mayor

biceps, bíceps

triceps brachii,
tríceps braquial

external oblique,
oblicuo externo

rectus abdominis,
recto del abdomen

gluteus maximus,
glùteo mayor

sartorius, sartorio
rectus femoris, recto femoral
vastus lateralis, vasto lateral

biceps femoris,
bíceps femoral

gastrocnemius, gemelos

Achilles tendon,
tendón de Aquiles

THE REPRODUCTIVE SYSTEM-EL SISTEMA REPRODUCTOR

The reproductive system, El sistema reproductor,

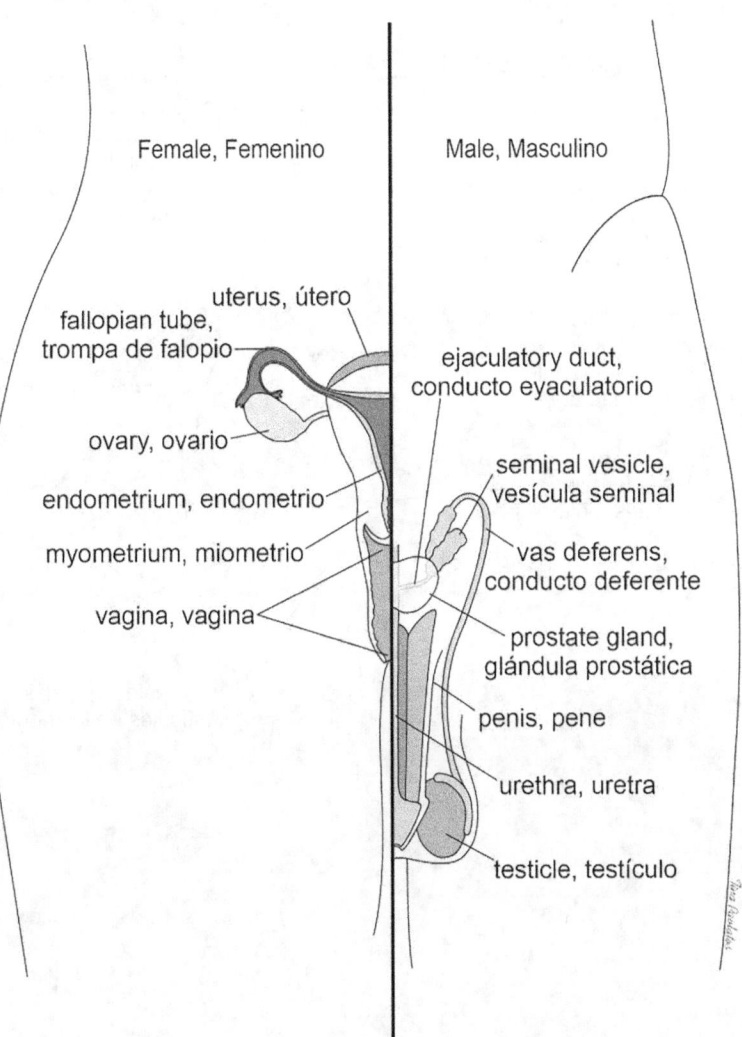

Female, Femenino

Male, Masculino

uterus, útero
fallopian tube,
trompa de falopio

ejaculatory duct,
conducto eyaculatorio

ovary, ovario

seminal vesicle,
vesícula seminal

endometrium, endometrio

myometrium, miometrio

vas deferens,
conducto deferente

vagina, vagina

prostate gland,
glándula prostática

penis, pene

urethra, uretra

testicle, testículo

THE ENDOCRINE SYSTEM-EL SISTEMA ENDOCRINO

Endocrine system, Sistema endocrino

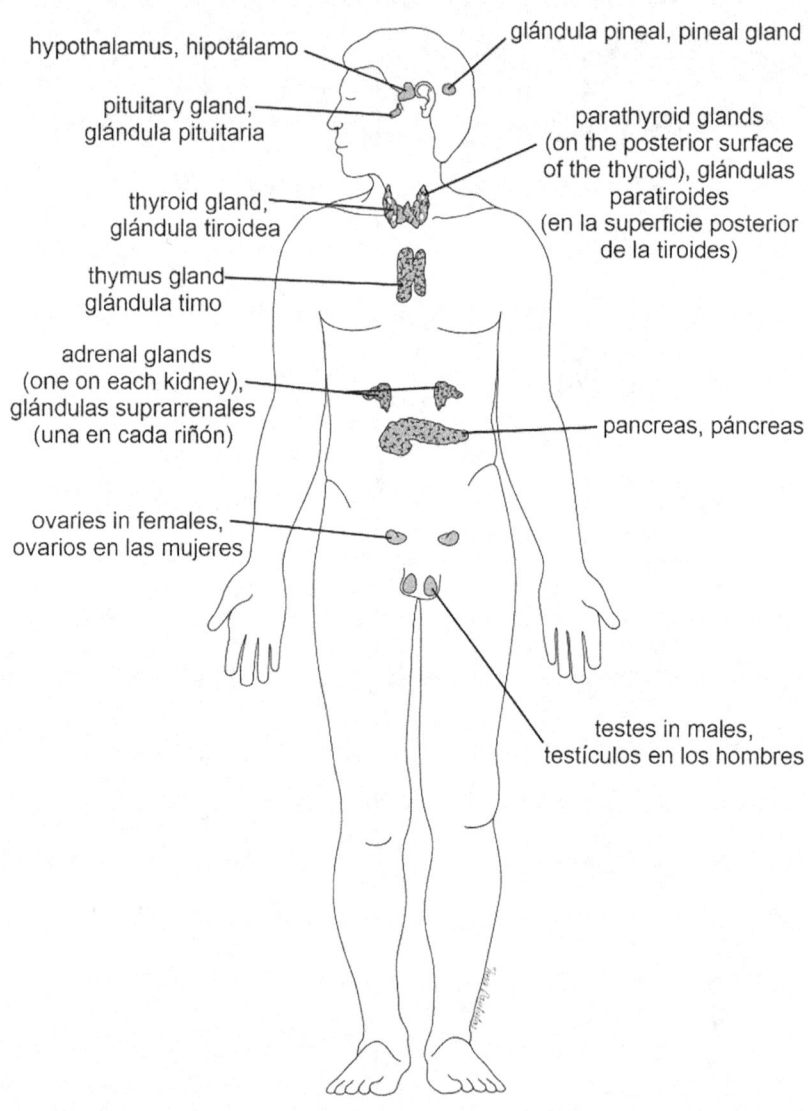

hypothalamus, hipotálamo

glándula pineal, pineal gland

pituitary gland, glándula pituitaria

parathyroid glands (on the posterior surface of the thyroid), glándulas paratiroides (en la superficie posterior de la tiroides)

thyroid gland, glándula tiroidea

thymus gland glándula timo

adrenal glands (one on each kidney), glándulas suprarrenales (una en cada riñón)

pancreas, páncreas

ovaries in females, ovarios en las mujeres

testes in males, testículos en los hombres

THE EYE-EL OJO

Eye, Ojo

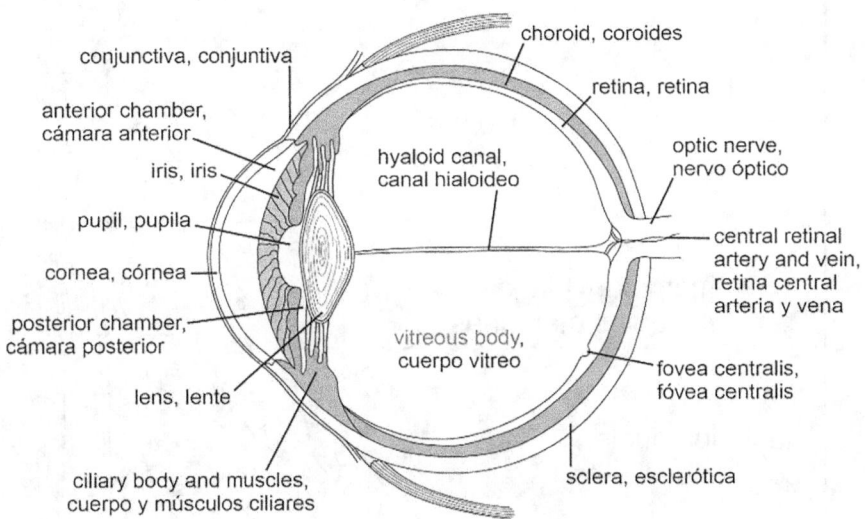

conjunctiva, conjuntiva

anterior chamber,
cámara anterior

iris, iris

pupil, pupila

cornea, córnea

posterior chamber,
cámara posterior

lens, lente

ciliary body and muscles,
cuerpo y músculos ciliares

choroid, coroides

retina, retina

hyaloid canal,
canal hialoideo

optic nerve,
nervo óptico

central retinal
artery and vein,
retina central
arteria y vena

vitreous body,
cuerpo vitreo

fovea centralis,
fóvea centralis

sclera, esclerótica

THE BREAST-EL SENO (LA MAMA)

The breast, El seno (la mama)

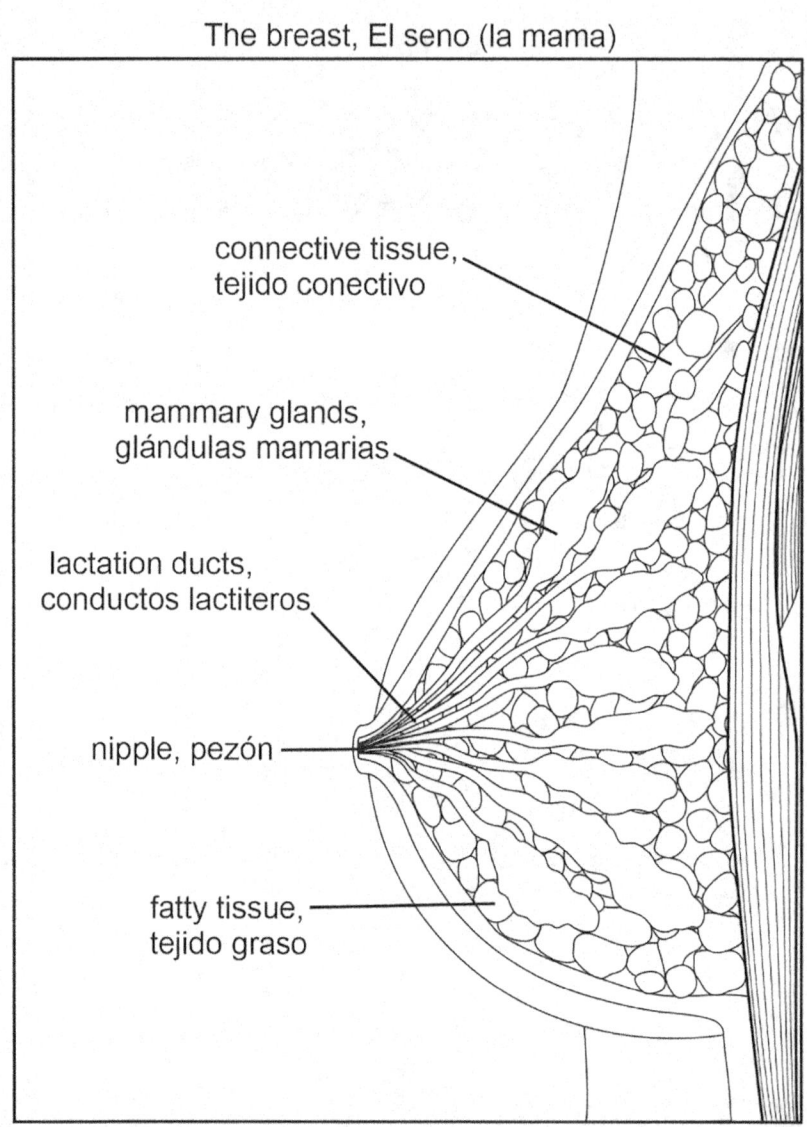

connective tissue, tejido conectivo

mammary glands, glándulas mamarias

lactation ducts, conductos lactiteros

nipple, pezón

fatty tissue, tejido graso

THE TEETH-LOS DIENTES

The teeth, Los dientes

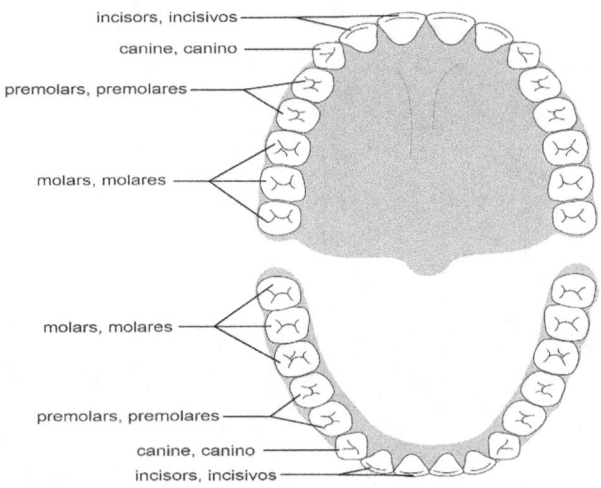

incisors, incisivos
canine, canino
premolars, premolares
molars, molares

molars, molares
premolars, premolares
canine, canino
incisors, incisivos

Tooth anatomy, Anatomía del diente

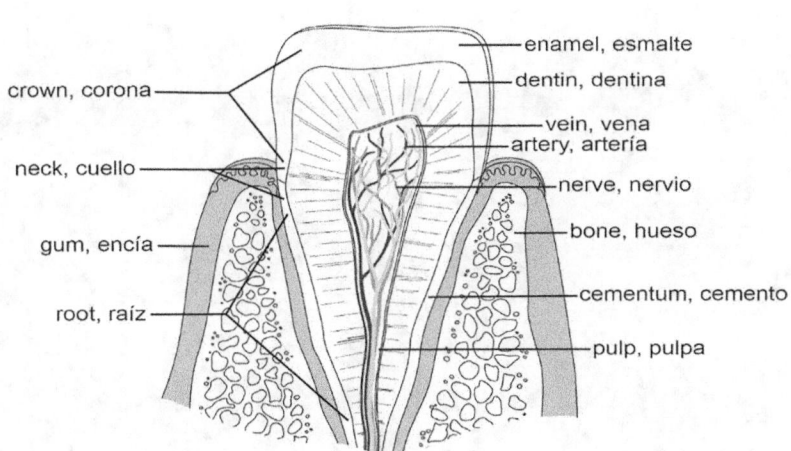

crown, corona
neck, cuello
gum, encía
root, raíz

enamel, esmalte
dentin, dentina
vein, vena
artery, artería
nerve, nervio
bone, hueso
cementum, cemento
pulp, pulpa

WORKBOOK

La cabeza. Please label each part of the head using the below word bank.

el paladar, el pelo/el cabello, los labios, las amígdalas, la pupila/la niña del ojo, la garganta, el cuero cabelludo, la lengua, el diente, los pómulos, el tabique, el párpado, la pestaña, el seno, la córnea, el mentón/la barbilla, las narices/las ventanas de la nariz, la fosa nasal, la ceja, el iris

The head, La cabeza

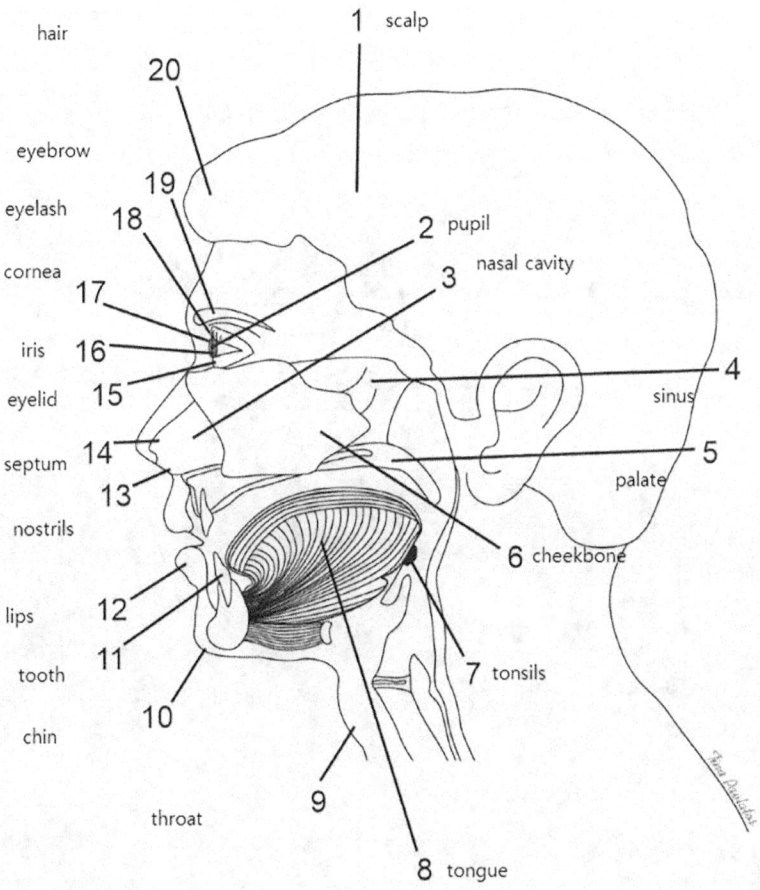

hair

1 scalp

20

eyebrow

19

eyelash

18

2 pupil

cornea

3 nasal cavity

17

iris 16

eyelid 15

4

sinus

septum 14

5

13

palate

nostrils

6 cheekbone

lips 12

11

7 tonsils

tooth

chin

10

throat

9

8 tongue

La boca Please label each part of the mouth using the below word bank.

La lengua, el labio superior, el arco palatofaríngeo, el paladar duro, la úvula, la encía, la amígdala palatina, el frenillo labial superior, el rafe palatino, el orofaringe, el arco palatoglosal, el frenillo lingual, el labio inferior, el paladar blando,el frenillo labia inferior, el vestíbulo, los conductos de la glándula submandibular

Mouth, Boca

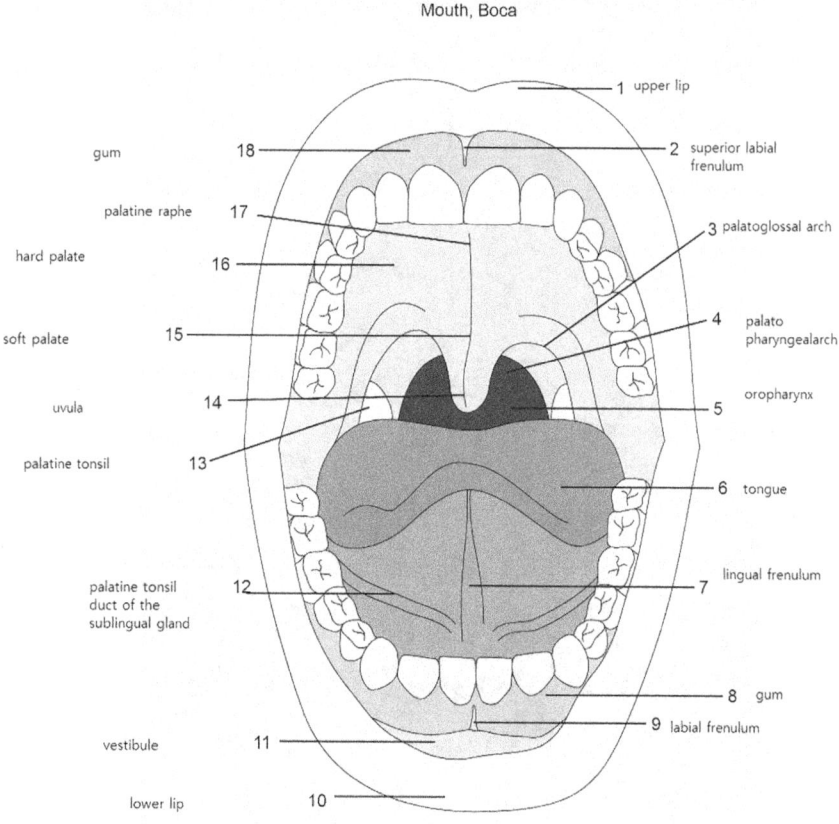

El cuerpo humano- Please label the body parts in Spanish using the attached word bank.

La barbilla/el mentón, la mejilla, el tobillo, la pantorilla, la muñeca, el brazo, el talón, el dedo del pie, el hombro, el dedo, el antebrazo, el codo, la rodilla, el pulgar, el pie, el pecho, el cuello, la boca, la cadera, la cabeza, la oreja, la nariz, los labios, la pierna, la frente, el ojo , el estómago, la palma, el oído, la ceja, la espinilla, el ombligo, la mano

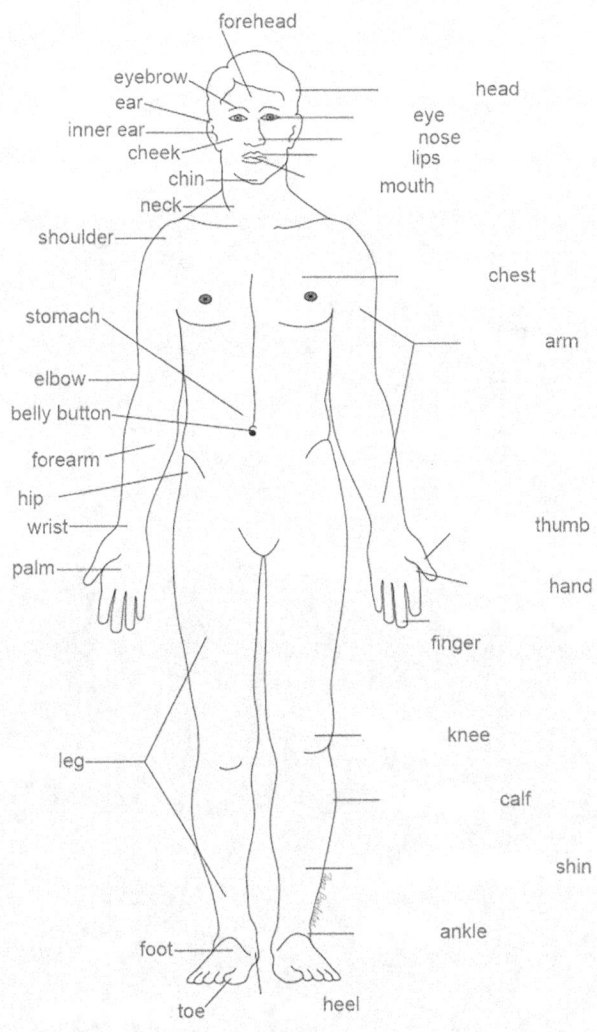

forehead

eyebrow
ear
inner ear
cheek
chin
neck

head
eye
nose
lips
mouth

shoulder

stomach

elbow

belly button

forearm

hip
wrist

palm

chest

arm

thumb

hand

finger

knee

calf

shin

ankle

leg

foot

toe   heel

El corazón. Please label each part of the heart using the below word bank.

> aorta descendente, válvulas, arteria aorta, ventrículo izquierdo, vena cava superior, aurícula derecha, vena cava inferior, ventrículo derecho, arteria pulmonar, aurícula izquierda, venas pulmonares

The heart, El corazón

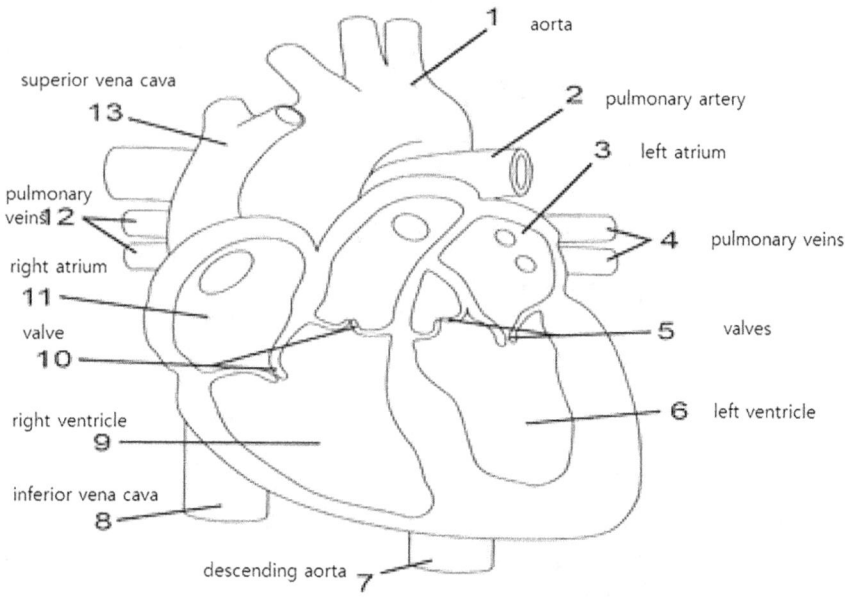

1 aorta
superior vena cava
13
2 pulmonary artery
3 left atrium
pulmonary veins 12
4 pulmonary veins
right atrium
11
valve
10
5 valves
6 left ventricle
right ventricle
9
inferior vena cava
8
descending aorta 7

El sistema circulatorio. .Please label each part of the circulatory system using the below word bank.

Vena cava superior, el corazón, aorta, vena safena interna, arteria pulmonar, arteria subclavia, , arteria carótida, vena yugular, arteria braquial, vena cava inferior, arteria femoral, vena subclavia, arteria radial, vena femoral, vena ilíaca, arteria ilíaca

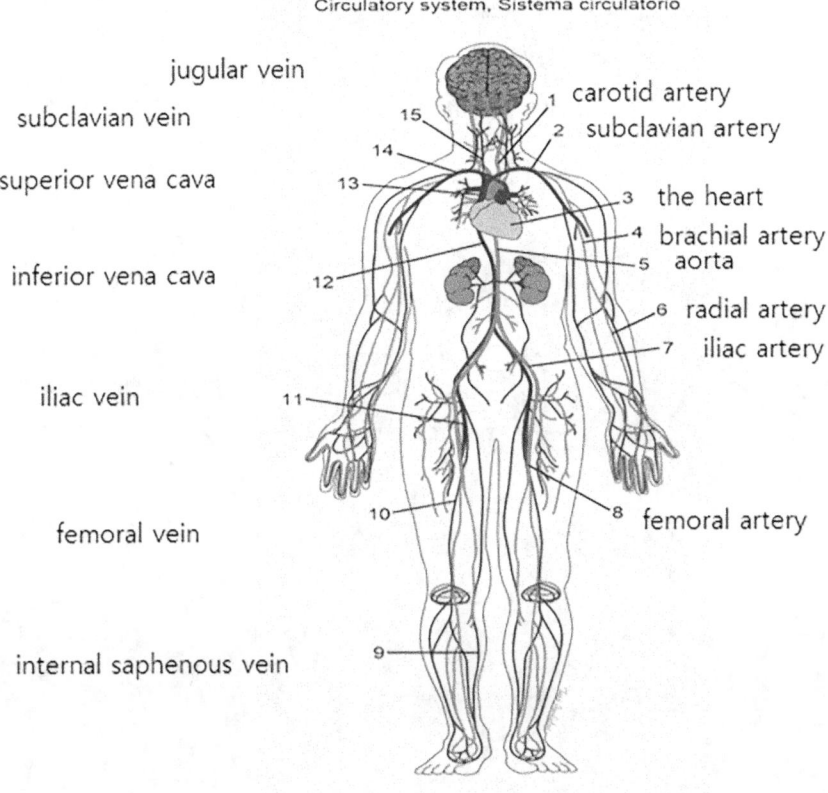

Circulatory system, Sistema circulatorio

jugular vein

subclavian vein

superior vena cava

inferior vena cava

iliac vein

femoral vein

internal saphenous vein

15
14
13
12
11
10
9

1 carotid artery
2 subclavian artery
3 the heart
4 brachial artery
5 aorta
6 radial artery
7 iliac artery
8 femoral artery

El sistema nervioso. Please label the nervous system in Spanish using the attached word bank.

Nervio tibial, encéfalo, nervio radial, nervio femoral, cerebelo, nervio cubital, médula espinal, nervios intercostales, nervio ciático, nervio peroneo

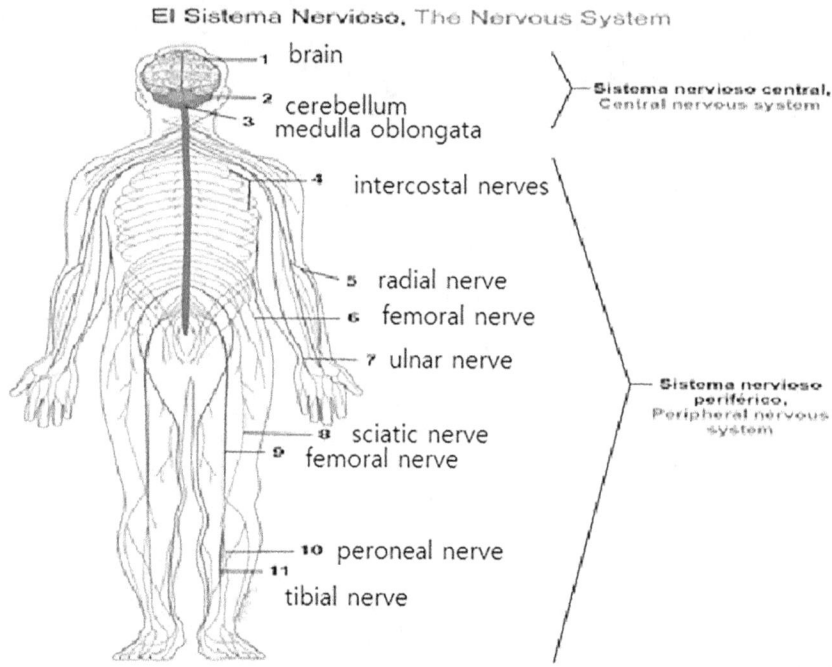

El Sistema Nervioso. The Nervous System

1 brain
2 cerebellum
3 medulla oblongata

Sistema nervioso central.
Central nervous system

4 intercostal nerves

5 radial nerve
6 femoral nerve
7 ulnar nerve

8 sciatic nerve
9 femoral nerve

Sistema nervioso
periférico.
Peripheral nervous
system

10 peroneal nerve
11 tibial nerve

El aparato digestivo. Please label the digestive system in Spanish using the attached word bank.

El ano, el hígado,el duodeno, el intestino grueso, las glándulas salivales, el intestino delgado, el conducto biliar, el estómago, el recto, el faringe, la boca, el esófago, la vesícula biliar, el apéndice,el páncreas

Digestive system, Aparato digestivo

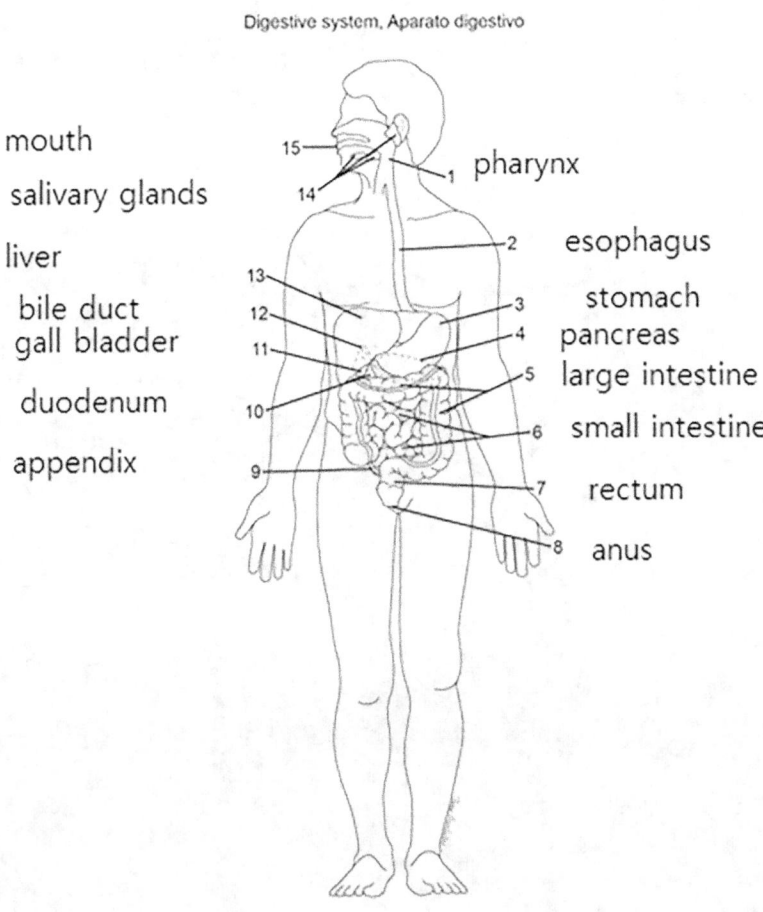

mouth

salivary glands

liver

  bile duct
  gall bladder

duodenum

appendix

15 —
14 —
13 —
12 —
11 —
10 —
9 —

1 pharynx

2 esophagus

3 stomach
4 pancreas
5 large intestine

6 small intestine

7 rectum

8 anus

El sistema respiratorio. Please label the respiratory system in Spanish using the attached word bank.

Las costillas, la fosa nasal, los centros respiratorios, los bronquios, el laringe, la cavidad abdominal, los músculos intercostales, la tráquea, la cavidad torácica, el faringe, el diafragma, el pulmón, las membranas pleurales, los bronquiolos

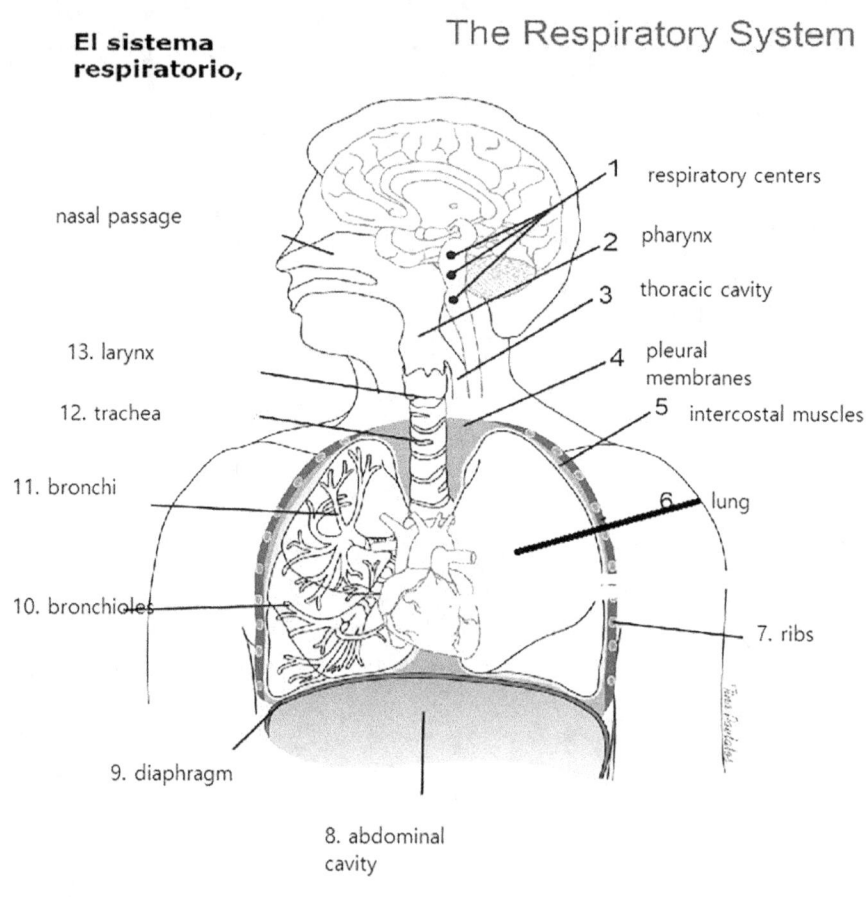

El sistema respiratorio,

The Respiratory System

1 respiratory centers

nasal passage

2 pharynx

3 thoracic cavity

13. larynx

4 pleural membranes

12. trachea

5 intercostal muscles

11. bronchi

6 lung

10. bronchioles

7. ribs

9. diaphragm

8. abdominal cavity

El sistema esquelético. Please label the skeletal system in Spanish using the attached word bank.

El pelvis, los metacarpianos el cúbito, los metatarsianos, la tibia, la escápula, la radio, los tarsales, el húmero, el peroné, la mandíbula, los carpos, las costillas, la rótula, el cráneo, falanges, la clavícula, vertebras, el fémur, el esternón

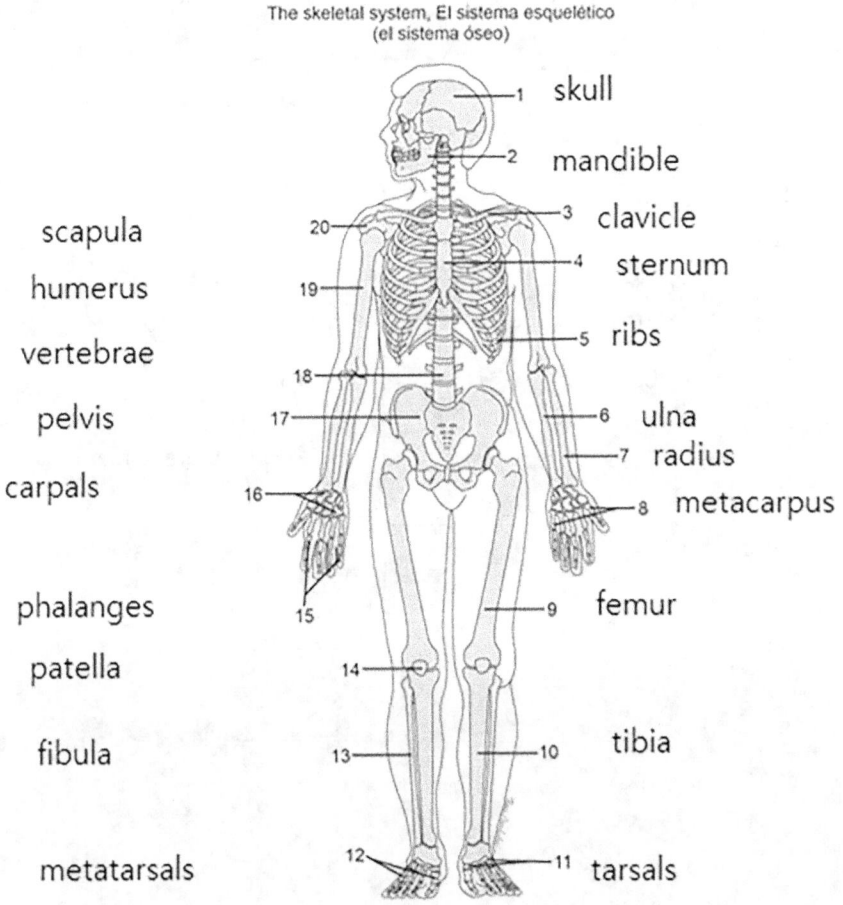

The skeletal system, El sistema esquelético
(el sistema óseo)

scapula
humerus
vertebrae
pelvis
carpals
phalanges
patella
fibula
metatarsals

1 skull
2 mandible
3 clavicle
4 sternum
5 ribs
6 ulna
7 radius
8 metacarpus
9 femur
10 tibia
11 tarsals

El sistema muscular. Please label the muscular system in Spanish using the attached word bank.

el Tendón de Aquiles, el pectoral mayor, el recto del abdomen, el masetero, los gemelos, el glúteo mayor, el sartorio, el esternocleidomastoideo, los bíceps, el recto femoral, el vasto lateral, el oblicuo externo, el trapecio, los triceps braquial, los biceps femoral

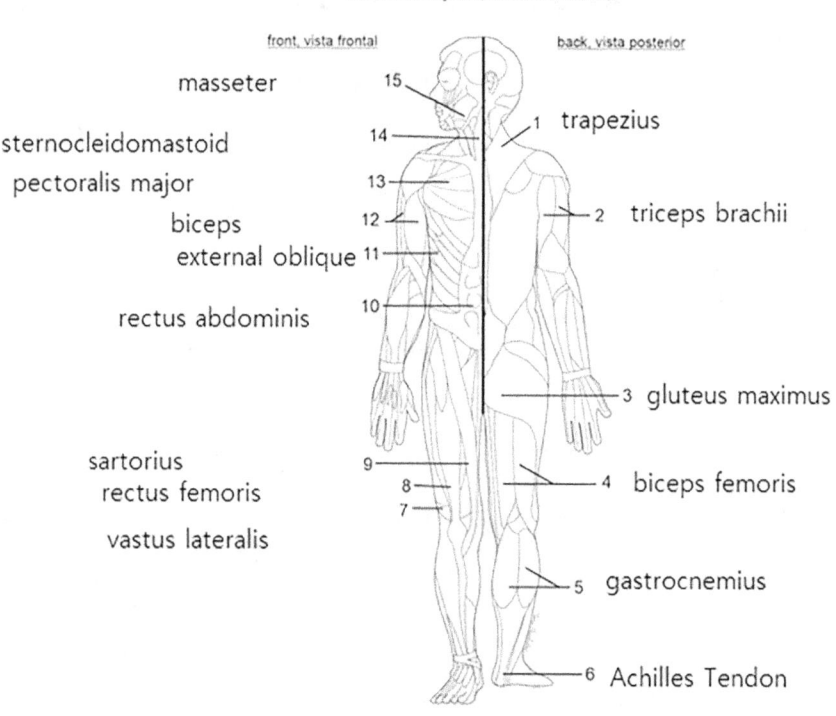

The muscular system. El sistema muscular

front, vista frontal   back, vista posterior

masseter   15

sternocleidomastoid   14   1 trapezius

pectoralis major   13

biceps   12   2 triceps brachii

external oblique   11

rectus abdominis   10

3 gluteus maximus

sartorius   9

rectus femoris   8   4 biceps femoris

7

vastus lateralis

5 gastrocnemius

6 Achilles Tendon

El sistema reproductor. Please label the reproductive system in Spanish using the attached word bank.

La uretra, el útero, la vagina, el conducto eyaculatorio, el pene, el testículo, el miometrio, la glándula prostática, el conducto deferente, la trompa de falopio, el ovario, el endometrio, la vesícula seminal

The reproductive system, El sistema reproductor,

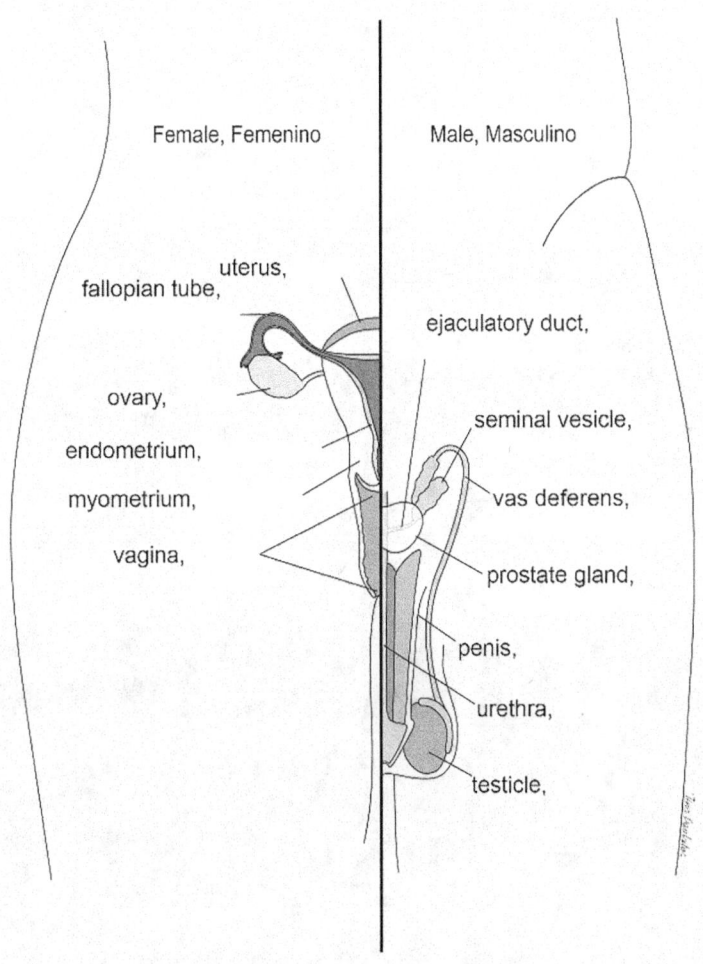

El sistema endocrino. Please label the endocrine system in Spanish using the attached word bank.

---

testículos, glándula timo, glándula pineal, glándula tiroidea, ovarios , páncreas,hipotálamo, glándulas paratiroides, glándulas suprarenales, glándula pituitaria

---

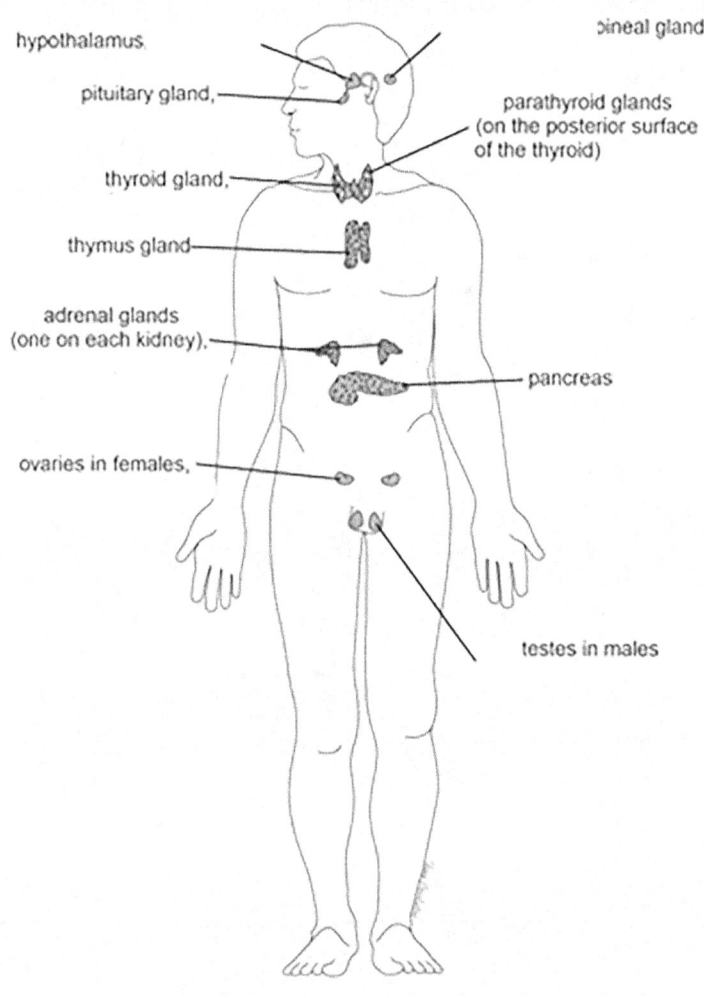

Endocrine system, Sistema endocrino

hypothalamus

pituitary gland,

thyroid gland,

thymus gland

adrenal glands
(one on each kidney),

ovaries in females,

pineal gland

parathyroid glands
(on the posterior surface
of the thyroid)

pancreas

testes in males

El ojo. Please label each part of the eye using the word bank.

lente, coroides, cámara anterior, retina, la córnea, pupila, nervio óptico, cuerpo vitreo, fovea centralis, retina central arteria y vena, esclerática, conjuntiva, cuerpo y músculos ciliares, cámara posterior,iris, canal hialoideo

Eye, Ojo

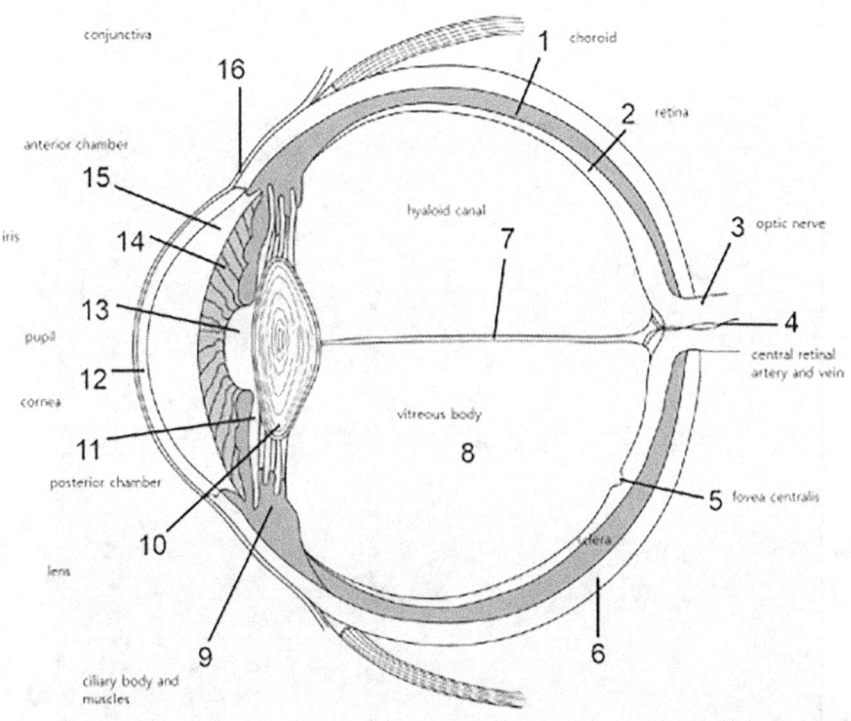

La mama. Please label the breast in Spanish using the attached word bank.

el pezón, las glándulas mamarias, el tejido conectivo, el tejido graso, los conductos lactiteros

The breast, El seno (la mama)

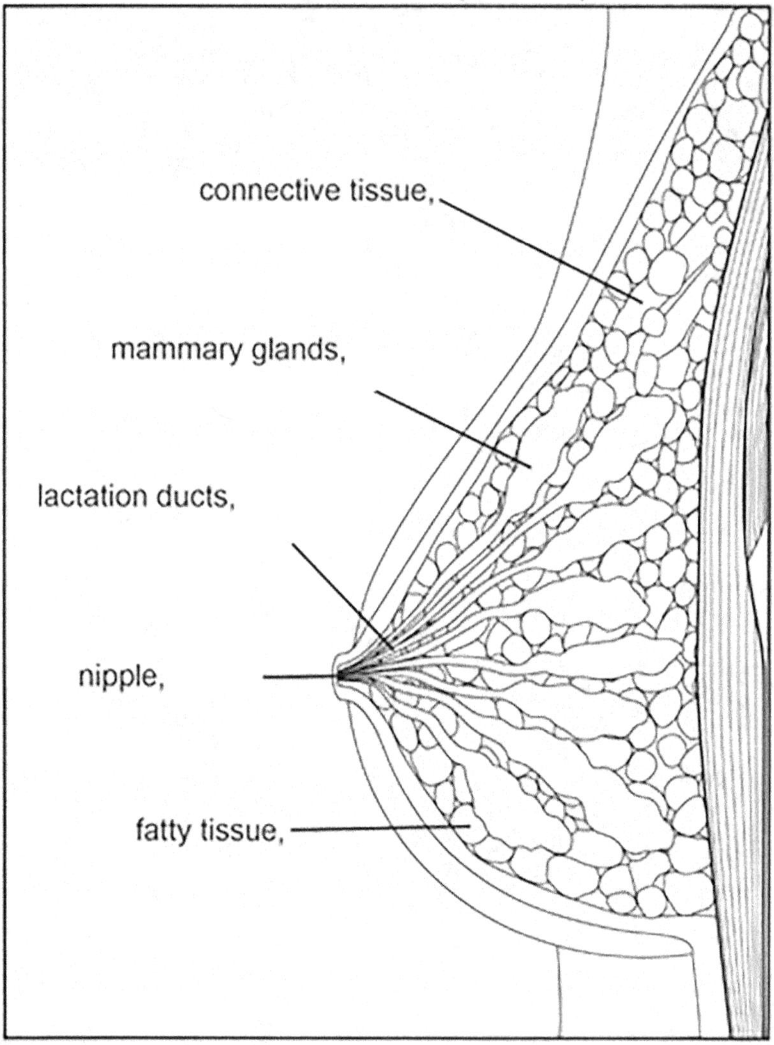

connective tissue,

mammary glands,

lactation ducts,

nipple,

fatty tissue,

THE TEETH Please pick the correct word from the wordbank.

The teeth. Los dientes

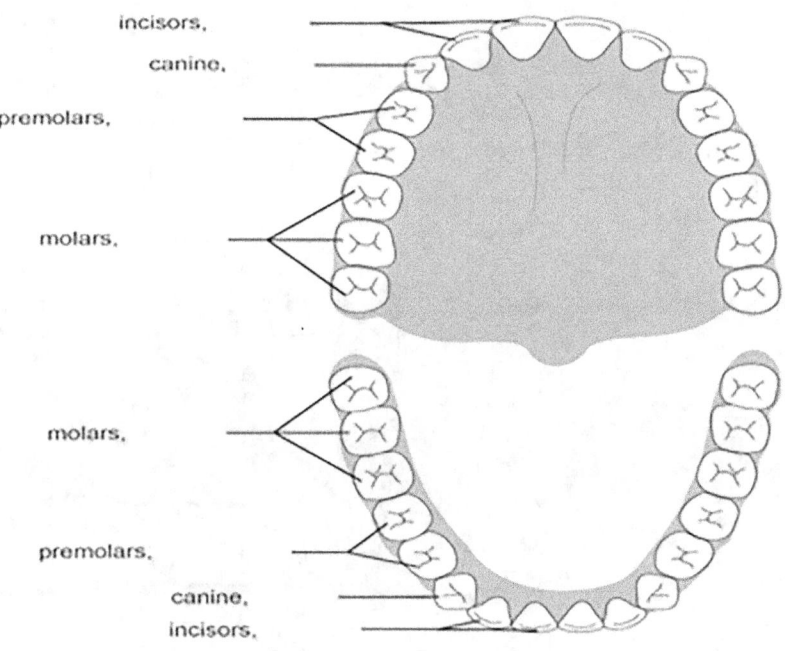

incisors,

canino,

premolars,

molars,

molars,

premolars,

canine,
incisors,

THE ANATOMY OF THE TOOTH Please pick the correct word from the wordbank.

El cemento, la corona, la pulpa, raíz, el hueso, la vena, el esmalte, la encía, el nervio, la vena, el cuello, la dentina, la artería

Tooth anatomy, Anatomía del diente

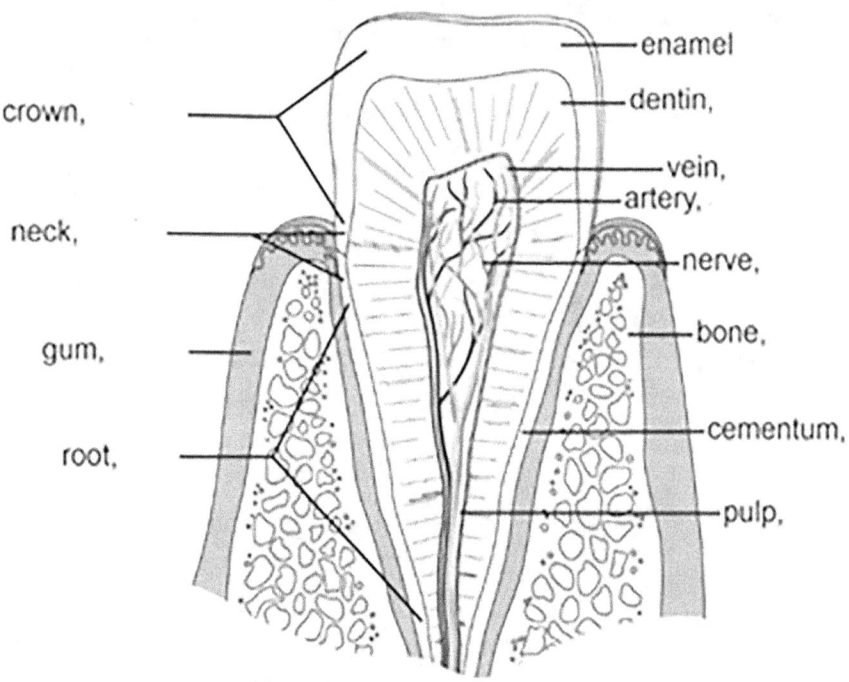

crown,

neck,

gum,

root,

enamel

dentin,

vein,

artery,

nerve,

bone,

cementum,

pulp,

ANSWER KEYS

The head, La cabeza

1. scalp, el cuero cabelludo
2. pupil, la pupila/la niña del ojo
3. nasal cavity, la fosa nasal
4. sinus, el seno
5. palate, el paladar
6. cheekbone, los pómulos
7. tonsils, las amígdalas/las anginas
8. tongue, la lengua
9. throat, la garganta
10. chin, el mentón/la barbilla
11. tooth, el diente
12. lips, los labios
13. nostrils, las narices/las ventanas de la nariz
14. septum, el tabique
15. eyelid, el párpado
16. iris, el iris
17. cornea, la córnea
18. eyelash, la pestaña
19. eyebrow, la ceja
20. hair, el pelo, el cabello

Mouth, Boca

1. upper lip, labio superior
2. superior labial frenulum, frenillo labial superior
3. palatoglossal arch, palatoglosal
4. palato pharyngealarch, palatofaríngeo
5. oropharynx, orofaringe
6. tongue, lengua
7. lingual frenulum, frenillo lingual
8. gum, encía
9. labial frenulum, frenillo labia inferior
10. lower lip, labio inferior
11. vestibule, vestíbulo
12. palatine tonsil duct of the sublingual gland, conductos de la glándula submandibular
13. palatine tonsil, amígdala palatina
14. uvula, úvula
15. soft palate, paladar blando
16. hard palate, paladar duro
17. alatine raphe, afe palatino
18. gum, encia

THE HUMAN BODY-EL CUERPO HUMANO

1. la frente, forehead	17. el dedo del pie, toe
2. la cabeza, head	18. el pie, foot
3. el ojo, eye	19. la pierna, leg
4. la nariz, nose	20. la palma, palm
5. los labios, lips	21. la muñeca, wrist
6. la boca, mouth	22. la cadera, hip
7. el pecho, chest	23. el antebrazo, forearm
8. el brazo, arm	24. el ombligo, belly button
9.el pulgar, thumb	25. el codo, elbow
10.la mano, hand	26. estómago, stomach
11. el dedo (el muslo), finger	27. el hombro, shoulder
	28. el cuello, neck
12. la rodilla, knee	29. la barbilla (el mentón), chin
13. la pantorrilla, calf	
14. la espinilla (la canilla), shin	30. la mejilla, cheek
	31. el oído, inner ear
15. el tobillo, ankle	32. la oreja, ear
16. el talón, heel	33. la ceja, eyebrow

El corazón, The heart

1. arteria aorta ,aorta
2. arteria pulmonar, pulmonary artery
3. aurícula izquierda, left atrium
4. venas pulmonares, pulmonary veins
5. válvulas, valves
6. ventrículo izquierdo, left ventricle

7. aorta descendente, descending aorta
8. vena cava inferior, inferior vena cava
9. ventriculo derecho, right ventricle
10. válvulas, valves
11. aurícula derecha, right atrium
12. venas pulmonares, pulmonary veins
13. vena cava superior, superior vena cava

THE CIRCULATORY SYSTEM .EL SISTEMA CIRCULATORIO ANSWER KEY

The Circulatory System   El sistema circulatorio

1. carotid artery, arteria carótida,
2. subclavian artery, arteria subclavia
3. the heart, el corazón
4. brachial artery, arteria braquial
5. aorta, aorta
6. radial artery, arteria radial
7. iliac artery, arteria ilíaca,
8. femoral artery, arteria femoral
9. internal saphenous vein, vena safena interna
10. femoral vein, vena femoral
11. iliac vein, vena ilíaca
12. inferior vena cava, vena cava inferior
13. superior vena cava, vena cava superior,
14. subclavian vein, vena subclavia
15. jugular vein, vena jugular

The nervous system, El sistema nervioso

Central nervous system, Sistema nervioso central

1. brain, encéfalo
2. cerebellum, cerebelo
3. medulla oblongata, médula espinal

Peripheral nervous system, Sistema nervioso periférico

4. intercostal nerves, nervios intercostales
5. radial nerve, nervio radial
6. femoral nerve, nervio femoral
7. ulnar nerve, nervio cubital
8. sciatic nerve, nervio ciático
9. femoral nerve, nervio femoral
10. peroneal nerve, nervio peroneo
11. tibial nerve, nervio tibial

Digestive system, Aparato digestivo

1. pharynx, faringe
2. esophagus, esófago
3. stomach, estómago
4. pancreas, páncreas
5. large intestine, intestino grueso
6. small intestine, intestino delgado
7. rectum, recto
8. anus, ano
9. appendix, apéndice
10. duodenum, duodeno
11. gall bladder, vesícula biliar
12. bile duct, conducto biliar
13. liver, hígado
14. salivary glands, glándulas salivales
15. mouth, boca

The respiratory system, El sisterna respiratorio

1. respiratory centers, centros respiratorios
2. pharynx, faringe
3. thoracic cavity, cavidad torácica
4. pleural membranes, membranas pleurales
5. intercostal muscles, músculos intercostales
6. lung, pulmón
7. ribs, costillas
8. abdominal cavity, cavidad abdominal
9. diaphragm, diafragma
10. bronchioles, bronquiolos
11. bronchi, bronquios
12. trachea, tráquea
13. larynx, laringe
14. nasal passage, fosa nasal

The skeletal system, El sistema esquelético, (el sistema óseo)

1. skull, cráneo
2. mandible, mandíbula
3. clavicle, clavicula
4. sternum, esternón
5. ribs, costillas
6. ulna, cúbito
7. radius, radio
8. metacarpus, metacarpianos
9. femur, fémur
10. tibia, tibia
11. tarsals, tarsales
12. metatarsals, metatarsianos
13. fibula, peroné
14. patella, rótula
15. phalanges, falanges
16. carpals, carpos
17. pelvis, pelvis
18. vertebrae, vertebras
19. humerus, húmero
20. scapula, escápula

The muscular system, El sistema muscular

<u>back, vista posterior</u>

1. trapezius, trapecio
2. triceps brachii, tríceps braquial
3. gluteus maximus, glùteo mayor
4. biceps femoris, bíceps femoral
5. gastrocnemius, gemelos
6. Achilles tendon, tendón de Aquiles

<u>front, vista frontal</u>

7. vastus lateralis, vasto lateral
8. rectus femoris, recto femoral
9. sartorius, sartorio
10. rectus abdominis, recto del abdomen
11. external oblique, oblicuo externo
12. biceps, bíceps
13. pectoralis major, pectoral mayor
14. sternocleidomastoid, esternocleidomastoideo
15. masseter, masetero

The reproductive system, El sistema reproductor

Female, Femenino

1. uterus, útero
2. fallopian tube, trompa de falopio
3. ovary, ovario
4. endometrium, endometrio
5. myometrium, miometrio
6. vagina, vagina

Male, Masculino

1. ejaculatory duct, conducto eyaculatorio
2. seminal vesicle, vesícula seminal
3. vas deferens, conducto deferente
4. prostate gland, glándula prostática
5. penis, pene
6. urethra, uretra
7. testicle, testículo

Endocrine system, Sistema endocrino

1. pineal gland, glándula pineal
2. parathyroid glands (on the posterior surface of the thyroid), glándulas paratiroides (en la superficie posterior de la tiroides)
3. pancreas, páncreas
4. testes in males, testículos en los hombres
5. ovaries in females, ovarios en las mujeres

6. adrenal glands (one on each kidney), glándulas suprarrenales (una en cada riñón)
7. thymus gland, glándula timo
8. thyroid gland, glándula tiroidea
9. pituitary gland, glándula pituitaria
10. hypothalamus, hipotálamo

Eye, Ojo

1. choroid, coroides
2. retina, retina
3. optic nerve, nervo óptico
4. central retinal artery and vein, retina central arteria y vena,
5. fovea centralis, fóvea centralis
6. sclera, esclerótica
7. hyaloid canal, canal hialoideo
8. vitreous body, cuerpo vitreo
9. ciliary body and muscles, cuerpo y músculos ciliares
10. lens, lente
11. posterior chamber, cámara posterior
12. cornea, córnea
13. pupil, pupila
14. iris, iris
15. anterior chamber, cámara anterior
16. conjunctiva, conjuntiva

The breast, El seno (la mama)

1. connective tissue, tejido conectivo
2. mammary glands, glándulas mamarias
3. lactation ducts, conductos lactiteros
4. nipple, pezón
5. fatty tissue, tejido graso

Los dientes, The teeth

1. incisivos, incisors
2. canino, canine
3. premolares, premolars
4. molares, molars
5. molares, molars
6. premolares, premolars
7. canino, canine
8. incisivos, incisors

Tooth anatomy, Anatomía del diente

1. enamel, esmalte
2. dentin, dentina
3. vein, vena
4. artery, artería
5. nerve, nervio
6. bone, hueso
7. cementum, cemento
8. pulp, pulpa
9. root, raíz
10. gum, encía
11. neck, cuello
12. crown, corona